Testosterone Factor

Your Path to Reclaiming Energy, Confidence, and Vitality

Dr. Maxwell G. C. Philip

TABLE OF CONTENTS

Introduction to Testosterone

Testosterone is a hormone that plays a crucial role in the development, health, and well-being of both men and women, although it's most commonly associated with men due to its impact on male physical characteristics and reproductive health. This hormone affects many aspects of life, from muscle mass and bone density to mood and energy levels. In recent years, the role of testosterone in overall health has become a focal point for researchers, health professionals, and the general public, leading to a better understanding of its functions and its importance beyond just sexual health.

Understanding Testosterone: The Basics

Testosterone is a hormone primarily produced in the testicles for men and in smaller amounts in the ovaries for women. It belongs to a class of hormones called androgens, which are sometimes referred to as "male hormones." However, testosterone is also important in the female body, where it contributes to muscle strength, bone density, and libido, among other functions.

The production of testosterone is regulated by the hypothalamus and pituitary gland in the brain. This process is part of a feedback loop called the hypothalamic-pituitary-gonadal (HPG) axis. The hypothalamus releases gonadotropin-releasing hormone (GnRH), which prompts the pituitary gland to secrete luteinizing hormone (LH) and follicle-stimulating hormone (FSH). These hormones then stimulate the testicles or ovaries to produce testosterone. Once the body senses enough testosterone is present, the hypothalamus and pituitary reduce their signals, maintaining a balanced level of testosterone in the bloodstream.

Functions of Testosterone:

- **Development of Male Characteristics:** Testosterone is responsible for the development of male characteristics during puberty, such as deepening of the voice, growth of facial and body hair, and increased muscle mass.
- **Reproductive Health:** Testosterone is essential for sperm production and libido in men, while in women, it also plays a role in sexual arousal and overall reproductive health.
- **Bone and Muscle Health:** Testosterone stimulates muscle protein synthesis, which helps in building muscle mass and maintaining bone density. This is particularly important for reducing the risk of osteoporosis.
- **Mental Health and Mood Regulation:** Testosterone influences mood and energy levels, often contributing to feelings of vitality and well-being. Low levels of testosterone have been associated with

symptoms like fatigue, irritability, and even depression.

- **Metabolic Health:** Testosterone plays a role in fat distribution and muscle mass, affecting body composition and metabolism. It can help maintain a lean body mass and regulate body fat distribution.

Why Testosterone Matters for Health and Well-being

Testosterone is much more than just a hormone for building muscle or influencing male characteristics; it's essential for both physical and mental well-being. Here are some reasons why testosterone is so important for health across the lifespan:

1. **Physical Vitality and Strength**
   Testosterone supports physical strength and endurance by enhancing muscle mass and bone density. Adequate levels of testosterone contribute to a leaner body composition, allowing people to maintain

muscle mass and reduce fat accumulation as they age. This is particularly important in men over the age of 30, when testosterone levels naturally begin to decline.

2. **Mental Clarity and Cognitive Health**
Testosterone is also linked to mental clarity, cognitive function, and emotional health. It can positively affect mood, motivation, and cognitive functions like memory and concentration. Studies have shown that low testosterone levels are sometimes correlated with memory issues and decreased focus, as well as symptoms of depression.

3. **Heart and Metabolic Health**
Testosterone has beneficial effects on heart health and metabolism, helping to regulate blood sugar levels, insulin sensitivity, and cholesterol levels. Maintaining healthy testosterone levels can lower the risk of metabolic syndrome, a cluster of conditions that increase the risk of heart disease, stroke, and diabetes.

4. **Emotional Resilience and Mood**
   Research shows a strong link between testosterone and mood regulation. Low testosterone levels can lead to mood swings, fatigue, and even depressive symptoms. On the other hand, adequate testosterone levels contribute to a sense of well-being, motivation, and emotional stability.

5. **Sexual Health and Libido**
   One of the primary functions of testosterone is regulating libido and sexual performance. Low testosterone levels can lead to decreased libido and, in some cases, erectile dysfunction in men. Women also experience libido fluctuations in relation to their testosterone levels, which can impact their sexual health and satisfaction.

6. **Aging and Longevity**
   Testosterone plays an essential role in maintaining physical and mental health as we age. By helping to preserve muscle mass, bone density, and cognitive

function, testosterone contributes to a healthier ageing process. In older adults, balanced testosterone levels have been linked to a better quality of life, lower rates of osteoporosis, and reduced risk of age-related diseases.

Myths and Facts About Testosterone

Testosterone is often misunderstood due to the numerous myths surrounding it. Here are some common myths about testosterone and the facts that dispel them:

Myth 1: Testosterone is Only Important for Men

Fact: While testosterone is the primary male sex hormone, it is also essential for women. In both genders, testosterone plays a vital role in muscle strength, bone density, energy levels, and libido. Women produce less testosterone than men, but the hormone is still essential for their overall health.

Myth 2: High Testosterone Levels Make You Aggressive

Fact: Testosterone has often been linked to aggressive or dominant behaviour, but research suggests that it does not necessarily cause aggression. Instead, testosterone influences motivation, assertiveness, and confidence. Aggressive behaviour is often more complex and influenced by numerous factors, including personality, environment, and upbringing.

Myth 3: Testosterone Boosters are a Quick Fix for Low Libido or Energy

Fact: While some supplements are marketed as "testosterone boosters," there is limited evidence to support the effectiveness of most over-the-counter options. True low testosterone levels require medical intervention, typically in the form of lifestyle adjustments or testosterone replacement therapy (TRT) under a healthcare provider's guidance.

Myth 4: More Testosterone Means Better Health

Fact: Excessive testosterone can actually be

harmful and lead to health issues like sleep apnea, cardiovascular problems, and an increased risk of blood clots. Testosterone levels must be balanced—too little or too much can negatively impact health. Optimal health is about maintaining appropriate levels, not just increasing testosterone levels indiscriminately.

Myth 5: Testosterone Decline Is an Inevitable Part of Aging

Fact: While testosterone levels tend to decline with age, lifestyle factors—such as diet, exercise, sleep, and stress management—can greatly influence testosterone production. Healthy lifestyle habits can help mitigate age-related testosterone decline, allowing individuals to maintain adequate hormone levels even as they age.

Myth 6: Testosterone Therapy is Dangerous and Unnecessary

Fact: Testosterone replacement therapy (TRT) can be a safe and effective treatment for those with clinically low testosterone levels. When supervised by a qualified healthcare provider,

TRT can help alleviate symptoms of low testosterone and improve quality of life. It is not necessary for everyone, and each person's situation should be carefully evaluated before considering TRT.

The Science Behind Testosterone

Testosterone is a powerful hormone that plays a central role in the development, maintenance, and regulation of several bodily systems. It's a key part of the endocrine system, which governs hormone production and distribution, impacting nearly every aspect of health. Understanding how testosterone is produced, how it influences physical and mental health, and how the endocrine system controls its release is essential for anyone looking to manage their health holistically.

How Testosterone is Produced in the Body

Testosterone production begins with a series of complex processes that start in the brain and ultimately lead to the release of testosterone from specific glands in the body. The pathway of testosterone production, known as the hypothalamic-pituitary-gonadal (HPG) axis, involves the brain, pituitary gland, and gonads (testes in men, ovaries in women).

1. **The Hypothalamus and Pituitary Gland**
   The process starts in the hypothalamus, a small region at the base of the brain. The hypothalamus releases a hormone called gonadotropin-releasing hormone (GnRH) in response to signals from the body indicating that testosterone levels need to be adjusted. GnRH travels to the pituitary gland, a pea-sized gland located just below the brain, stimulating it to release two other hormones: luteinizing hormone (LH) and follicle-stimulating hormone (FSH).
2. **The Role of Luteinizing Hormone (LH) and Follicle-Stimulating Hormone**

(FSH)

LH and FSH are critical players in testosterone production. LH is directly responsible for stimulating the Leydig cells in the testes (for men) and ovarian cells (for women) to produce testosterone. FSH, on the other hand, is primarily involved in the regulation of sperm production in men and the development of ovarian follicles in women.

3. **Testosterone Production in Men and Women**
    - **In Men**: Once LH reaches the testes, it activates the Leydig cells, leading to the synthesis and release of testosterone. Testosterone is then released into the bloodstream, where it travels to target tissues, including muscle, bone, and the reproductive organs.
    - **In Women**: While women produce much less testosterone, it is still essential for their health. In women, the ovaries, adrenal glands, and

peripheral tissues all contribute to testosterone production. In the ovaries, a small number of cells respond to LH by producing testosterone, which is later converted into oestrogen, the primary female sex hormone.

4. **Testosterone in the Bloodstream**
   Once produced, testosterone doesn't simply remain idle in the bloodstream. Most of it binds to proteins, specifically sex hormone-binding globulin (SHBG) and albumin, which carry testosterone to target tissues. A small percentage of testosterone remains "free," meaning it's unbound and able to enter cells directly to exert its effects. Free testosterone is considered the most bioavailable form and has the most direct impact on tissues.

Hormones and Their Role in Physical and Mental Health

Hormones are chemical messengers produced by glands in the endocrine system that regulate almost every bodily function, from metabolism and growth to mood and reproductive health. Testosterone is one of many hormones that influence physical and mental health, and it has specific functions essential for maintaining overall balance.

1. **Muscle and Bone Health**
   Testosterone promotes muscle protein synthesis, a process that helps build and maintain muscle tissue. It also plays a role in bone density by stimulating bone-forming cells, called osteoblasts, which prevent bone loss. This is one reason why men typically have higher bone density and muscle mass than women. For both genders, maintaining sufficient testosterone levels is essential for preventing muscle wasting and osteoporosis, especially with age.

2. **Mood and Cognitive Function**
   Testosterone has profound effects on mental health and cognitive function. It's been shown to influence neurotransmitters

like dopamine and serotonin, which regulate mood, energy levels, and motivation. Low levels of testosterone are associated with mood disorders, such as depression, anxiety, and irritability. Some studies also suggest that adequate testosterone levels can support cognitive functions, including memory, spatial awareness, and focus, which may decline with age as testosterone levels decrease.

3. **Libido and Sexual Health**
Testosterone is essential for sexual health in both men and women. In men, it regulates libido, erectile function, and overall sexual performance. In women, testosterone contributes to sexual arousal, sensitivity, and pleasure. Low testosterone levels in either gender can lead to reduced libido and sexual satisfaction, impacting relationships and self-esteem.

4. **Energy Levels and Metabolism**
Testosterone influences energy metabolism and helps regulate blood sugar and fat distribution. Higher levels of

testosterone are associated with increased muscle mass, which in turn raises the body's resting metabolic rate (RMR). This metabolic boost allows the body to burn more calories at rest, making it easier to maintain a healthy weight. Low testosterone levels can lead to fatigue and reduced energy expenditure, which may contribute to weight gain and decreased physical activity.

5. **Stress Response and Resilience**
Testosterone interacts with cortisol, the primary stress hormone. Balanced testosterone levels can help blunt the effects of cortisol, promoting a healthier stress response. When testosterone is low, cortisol's effects are more pronounced, leading to higher stress levels, reduced resilience, and possibly, mental health challenges.

The Endocrine System and Testosterone Regulation

The endocrine system is the network of glands that produce, regulate, and release hormones into the bloodstream. This system includes the hypothalamus, pituitary gland, thyroid, adrenal glands, pancreas, and gonads. The regulation of testosterone is one of many processes managed by this system, and it relies on a carefully balanced feedback loop that keeps testosterone levels within an optimal range.

1. **The Hypothalamic-Pituitary-Gonadal (HPG) Axis**

   As noted earlier, the HPG axis is the key pathway for testosterone production and regulation. When the hypothalamus detects low testosterone levels in the bloodstream, it releases GnRH to stimulate the pituitary gland. The pituitary gland then secretes LH and FSH, which prompt the gonads to produce more testosterone. If testosterone levels are high, the hypothalamus reduces GnRH production, slowing down the entire process and preventing excessive hormone levels.

2. **Negative Feedback Loop**

   Testosterone regulation is governed by a negative feedback loop, a mechanism that prevents the overproduction of hormones. When testosterone levels are sufficient, receptors in the hypothalamus and pituitary gland detect this and reduce the release of GnRH, LH, and FSH, decreasing testosterone production. This loop keeps testosterone within a balanced range, avoiding extreme fluctuations that could lead to health issues.

3. **Role of Sex Hormone-Binding Globulin (SHBG)**

   SHBG is a protein that binds to testosterone, controlling how much of the hormone is active and available in the body. When SHBG levels are high, more testosterone is bound and inactive, leading to lower bioavailable testosterone. Factors like ageing, lifestyle, and certain medical conditions can increase SHBG levels, reducing the amount of free testosterone and impacting its effectiveness.

4. **Impact of Other Hormones on Testosterone Levels**
   The endocrine system is highly interconnected, meaning that changes in one hormone can affect others. For example:
   - **Cortisol**: High levels of cortisol, often due to chronic stress, can inhibit testosterone production. Cortisol competes with testosterone, and sustained stress can lead to reduced testosterone levels over time.
   - **Insulin**: Insulin resistance, often associated with obesity, can lead to lower testosterone levels in men. Excessive insulin production can interfere with the HPG axis, reducing testosterone production.
   - **Oestrogen**: In men, high levels of oestrogen can suppress testosterone production. Some testosterone

naturally converts to oestrogen through a process called aromatization, and excess body fat can increase this conversion rate, leading to a reduction in testosterone levels.

5. **Age-Related Changes in Testosterone Regulation**

As people age, the body's ability to produce and regulate testosterone decreases. This decline is often gradual, with testosterone levels typically peaking in early adulthood and slowly declining around 1% per year after the age of 30. Ageing affects not only the production of testosterone in the gonads but also the sensitivity of the hypothalamus and pituitary to testosterone levels, which can disrupt the HPG axis. For many men, this decrease in testosterone levels may lead to symptoms associated with andropause, or "male menopause," including reduced energy, loss of muscle mass, and lower libido.

6. **Environmental and Lifestyle Influences on Testosterone Regulation**
   Factors like diet, exercise, sleep, and exposure to endocrine-disrupting chemicals (EDCs) can also impact the regulation of testosterone. A diet rich in nutrients, regular physical activity, and adequate sleep can promote healthy testosterone levels. In contrast, EDCs, which are found in certain plastics, pesticides, and personal care products, can interfere with hormone production and balance, potentially disrupting the endocrine system's ability to regulate testosterone.

Symptoms of Low Testosterone

Low testosterone, or "low T," affects many aspects of health, from physical fitness and sexual function to mood and mental well-being. Recognizing the signs of low testosterone early can help individuals seek effective treatment and lifestyle adjustments to mitigate the impact on their quality of life. Here, we'll examine the broad symptoms, as well as the specific ways low testosterone impacts physical, psychological, and emotional health.

Recognizing the Signs of Low Testosterone

The symptoms of low testosterone can vary widely depending on factors such as age, overall health, and lifestyle. Many symptoms are subtle at first, which means they may be overlooked or attributed to other causes like ageing or stress. Recognizing these early warning signs is essential for understanding and managing testosterone deficiency.

1. **Low Libido**

   One of the most noticeable and common signs of low testosterone is a reduced sex drive, or libido. Testosterone is a key hormone in sexual arousal and interest in both men and women, although its effects are more pronounced in men. A noticeable drop in sexual desire, especially if it's significantly different from one's normal level, can often be one of the first indicators of low testosterone.

2. **Erectile Dysfunction**

   In men, testosterone plays a critical role in achieving and maintaining erections. Although testosterone isn't solely responsible for erections—other factors, like blood flow and nerve function, are also involved—a deficiency can lead to weaker or less frequent erections, especially during spontaneous situations like sleep or early morning. Low testosterone can exacerbate erectile dysfunction (ED) caused by other factors, such as cardiovascular issues or diabetes.

3. **Fatigue and Reduced Energy Levels**
Feeling chronically tired and lacking energy, even with sufficient sleep, is a common symptom of low testosterone. The hormone is involved in energy metabolism, and low levels may lead to persistent fatigue that doesn't improve with rest. This fatigue can affect productivity, motivation, and the ability to stay active, creating a vicious cycle that further deteriorates physical health.

4. **Loss of Muscle Mass and Strength**
Testosterone is essential for muscle growth and maintenance, and a drop in testosterone levels can lead to a decrease in muscle mass and strength. Men with low testosterone may find it more challenging to build muscle, even with

regular exercise, and may notice a gradual loss of muscle tone over time. This loss of muscle can contribute to physical weakness, reduce metabolism, and increase the risk of injury.

5. **Increased Body Fat**
Low testosterone levels are associated with an increase in body fat, particularly around the abdomen. Testosterone helps regulate fat distribution, and without sufficient levels, fat tends to accumulate more easily. Additionally, lower testosterone may lead to increased levels of oestrogen, which can also contribute to fat storage. Increased body fat can worsen the effects of low testosterone, as fat cells contribute to the conversion of testosterone into oestrogen, creating a cycle of hormonal imbalance.

6. **Decreased Bone Density**
Testosterone is crucial for maintaining bone density, and low levels can lead to a decrease in bone mass, increasing the risk of osteoporosis and fractures. In severe

cases, men with low testosterone are at a higher risk for brittle bones, especially as they age. Bone density loss may go unnoticed until a fracture or other injury occurs, making it essential to address low testosterone early to prevent long-term damage.

7. **Hair Loss**

While hair loss is primarily genetic, testosterone plays a role in hair growth on both the scalp and body. Low testosterone may lead to hair thinning or a reduction in body and facial hair in men. Although this isn't a definitive symptom, sudden or noticeable changes in hair growth patterns may indicate low testosterone.

8. **Hot Flashes**

While typically associated with menopause, hot flashes can also be a symptom of low testosterone in men. They occur due to hormonal fluctuations and may include sweating, warmth in the upper body, and a sudden feeling of heat. This symptom is particularly noticeable in men undergoing testosterone replacement therapy but may also occur with naturally low testosterone levels.

How Low Testosterone Affects Physical Health

The physical impacts of low testosterone extend beyond the symptoms above, influencing overall health in ways that may increase the risk of other conditions. The following are some of the more specific ways low testosterone can affect physical well-being.

1. **Cardiovascular Health**

   Low testosterone is associated with an increased risk of cardiovascular diseases. Testosterone plays a role in red blood cell production and helps regulate cholesterol levels. Lower levels of testosterone may lead to a higher risk of conditions like high blood pressure, atherosclerosis, and heart attacks. Research indicates that men with low testosterone levels are more likely to experience cardiovascular events than those with adequate hormone levels.

2. **Insulin Resistance and Metabolic Syndrome**

   Testosterone has a role in regulating blood sugar levels and insulin sensitivity. Men with low testosterone are more likely to develop insulin resistance, a condition where the body doesn't respond effectively to insulin, leading to high blood sugar levels. Insulin resistance often progresses to metabolic syndrome—a cluster of conditions that include high blood pressure, high blood sugar, increased body fat, and abnormal cholesterol levels—which raises the risk of heart disease, stroke, and diabetes.

3. **Immune Function**

   Testosterone has a complex relationship with the immune system. While it generally has a mild suppressive effect on immune function, it is also crucial for reducing chronic inflammation. Low testosterone levels can lead to higher levels of inflammation, which can stress the immune system and increase susceptibility to illnesses.

4. **Physical Performance and Stamina**
   Testosterone impacts physical stamina and endurance, partly due to its effects on muscle mass and energy levels. Low testosterone can decrease physical performance and exercise capacity, making it harder to stay fit and active. Over time, this can lead to a sedentary lifestyle, which can worsen the symptoms associated with low testosterone and increase the risk of chronic health issues.

Psychological and Emotional Impacts of Low Testosterone

Beyond the physical symptoms, low testosterone can profoundly affect mental health, mood, and emotional well-being. This impact can sometimes be as significant as, or even more disruptive than, the physical effects.

1. **Mood Swings and Irritability**
   Men with low testosterone often report mood changes, including irritability and increased emotional sensitivity. Testosterone has an influence on neurotransmitters, such as serotonin and dopamine, which regulate mood and emotional responses. Low testosterone levels can disrupt these chemicals, leading to mood swings, irritability, and feelings of frustration.

2. **Depression and Anxiety**
   Low testosterone is linked with higher rates of depression and anxiety. This may be due to testosterone's effects on brain chemistry and its influence on the parts of the brain responsible for regulating mood. Studies show that men with lower testosterone levels are more prone to depressive symptoms, lack of motivation, and feelings of sadness. Treatment to increase testosterone levels can sometimes alleviate these symptoms and improve mental health outcomes.

3. **Reduced Self-Confidence and Self-Esteem**

   The physical symptoms of low testosterone, such as reduced muscle mass, increased body fat, and sexual dysfunction, can negatively impact self-image and confidence. When a person feels less physically capable or perceives themselves as less attractive, it can lead to lowered self-esteem. Over time, this can create a cycle of diminished confidence and motivation, which affects mental health and social interactions.

4. **Memory and Cognitive Impairment**

   Testosterone is thought to play a role in cognitive functions, including memory, attention, and processing speed. Research suggests that low testosterone can contribute to memory problems and cognitive decline, which may be partly due to the hormone's influence on blood flow and brain health. Low testosterone levels have been linked to conditions like brain fog and forgetfulness, which may impact daily functioning and productivity.

5. **Lack of Motivation and Drive**
Testosterone influences motivation, competitiveness, and drive. When testosterone levels are low, individuals may experience a loss of ambition and enthusiasm, sometimes described as a feeling of being "unmotivated." This lack of drive can impact both personal and professional life, potentially leading to missed opportunities, reduced productivity, and dissatisfaction with achievements.

6. **Social Withdrawal and Isolation**
Due to mood changes, lack of confidence, and reduced energy, people with low testosterone may become more socially withdrawn. Low testosterone can make social interactions feel less appealing or enjoyable, which can contribute to feelings of isolation and loneliness. Additionally, the stigma surrounding low testosterone and its effects on sexual

health can make it difficult for people to seek support from friends, family, or professionals.

Causes of Low Testosterone

Low testosterone, a condition known as hypogonadism, can result from various factors. While ageing is a natural cause, certain lifestyle choices, medical conditions, and environmental influences can also lead to reduced testosterone production. Understanding these causes can help individuals and healthcare providers develop strategies to maintain healthy testosterone levels and manage symptoms effectively.

Ageing and Its Effect on Testosterone Levels

As men age, it's natural for testosterone levels to gradually decline. This decrease usually begins around age 30 and continues at a rate of approximately 1% per year. By the time men reach their 50s, testosterone levels are significantly lower than in their youth, contributing to a range of age-related changes in physical, mental, and sexual health.

1. **Reduced Testosterone Production**
   The testicles and the hypothalamus, which together regulate testosterone production, become less effective with age. The Leydig cells in the testicles that produce testosterone begin to deteriorate, reducing the body's overall ability to synthesise this hormone. Aging can also lead to changes in the hypothalamus and pituitary gland, both of which play key roles in signalling the testes to produce testosterone.

2. **Increased Sex Hormone-Binding Globulin (SHBG)**
   As men age, levels of sex hormone-binding globulin (SHBG) tend to rise. SHBG binds to testosterone in the bloodstream, rendering it inactive. This increase in SHBG means that even if total testosterone levels remain relatively

stable, less of it is available for the body to use, leading to symptoms associated with low testosterone.

3. **Impact on Physical Health and Function**

   With age, the natural decline in testosterone can lead to decreased muscle mass, reduced bone density, increased body fat, and a decrease in overall energy. This process is sometimes referred to as "andropause," similar to menopause in women, though it occurs gradually over a longer period.

4. **Cognitive and Emotional Changes**

   The age-related decline in testosterone also contributes to cognitive changes, such as reduced mental sharpness and memory issues. Emotionally, it can lead to a loss of motivation, decreased confidence, and feelings of depression or anxiety. These cognitive and emotional shifts, coupled with physical symptoms, can significantly impact a man's quality of life.

5. **Sexual Health**

   Testosterone is essential for maintaining libido, erectile function, and overall sexual health. Age-related testosterone decline is commonly associated with decreased sexual desire and, in some cases, erectile dysfunction. While these changes may be gradual, they often become more pronounced as men reach their 50s and 60s.

Lifestyle Factors That Influence Testosterone

Several lifestyle choices can also influence testosterone levels, some of which are modifiable and can help individuals manage or prevent low testosterone.

1. **Diet and Nutrition**

   Poor dietary habits, particularly diets high in processed foods, refined sugars, and unhealthy fats, can negatively affect testosterone production. Diets lacking in essential nutrients like zinc, magnesium, and vitamin D are associated with lower testosterone levels, as these nutrients play key roles in testosterone synthesis. On the other hand, balanced diets rich in lean proteins, healthy fats, and vegetables can support healthy hormone levels.

2. **Physical Activity and Sedentary Lifestyle**

   Physical activity, particularly resistance and strength training, is beneficial for maintaining testosterone levels. Sedentary behaviour and prolonged inactivity, however, can lead to decreased testosterone. Excessive endurance exercise, like long-distance running, can also suppress testosterone, as it may increase cortisol levels, a stress hormone that can counteract testosterone production.

3. **Obesity**

   Excess body fat, particularly abdominal fat, is a major factor in low testosterone. Fat cells convert testosterone into oestrogen, the primary female sex hormone, leading to a further reduction in available testosterone. This increase in oestrogen can create a hormonal imbalance, leading to additional testosterone loss. Obesity is also linked with insulin resistance, which can impact overall metabolic health and contribute to low testosterone.

4. **Stress and Cortisol Levels**
Chronic stress elevates cortisol levels, which in turn can suppress testosterone production. Cortisol and testosterone have an inverse relationship, meaning that high cortisol levels reduce testosterone levels. Chronic stress from work, relationships, or personal challenges can contribute significantly to hormonal imbalances, and over time, it can lead to noticeable declines in testosterone.

5. **Sleep Patterns**
Quality sleep is crucial for testosterone production, as the body produces the majority of its testosterone during sleep, particularly during the REM phase. Poor sleep habits, such as insufficient sleep,

irregular sleep patterns, or sleep disorders like sleep apnea, can reduce testosterone levels. Studies show that men who sleep less than 5-6 hours per night are more likely to have lower testosterone levels than those who get adequate sleep.

6. **Alcohol and Substance Abuse**
Excessive alcohol consumption is linked to reduced testosterone levels. Alcohol affects the endocrine system and interferes with testosterone production, particularly in heavy drinkers. Alcohol's impact on the liver can also impair the body's ability to metabolise oestrogen, leading to higher levels of oestrogen in the bloodstream and reducing testosterone. Additionally, recreational drugs like marijuana can also lower testosterone, especially with frequent use.

Medical Conditions Linked to Low Testosterone

Various medical conditions can interfere with the body's ability to produce or regulate testosterone, either directly or indirectly.

1. **Hypogonadism**

   Hypogonadism is a condition in which the body's glands produce insufficient testosterone due to problems with the testicles or the pituitary gland. This condition can be congenital or develop later in life. Primary hypogonadism results from issues with the testicles themselves, while secondary hypogonadism is due to issues with the pituitary gland or hypothalamus, which control hormone production.

2. **Type 2 Diabetes**

   Type 2 diabetes is strongly linked to low testosterone. The insulin resistance associated with diabetes impacts hormone levels, often leading to lower testosterone in men. Low testosterone is also a risk factor for developing diabetes, as it influences body composition and fat distribution, both of which affect insulin sensitivity. The link between these two conditions is complex and often creates a cycle of declining health if left unaddressed.

3. **Metabolic Syndrome**
   Metabolic syndrome is a collection of conditions that increase the risk of heart disease, stroke, and diabetes, including high blood pressure, high blood sugar, excess abdominal fat, and abnormal cholesterol levels. Low testosterone is often seen in men with metabolic syndrome, and the presence of this condition may contribute to a further decline in testosterone due to increased body fat and other metabolic disruptions.

4. **Thyroid Disorders**
   The thyroid gland, which controls metabolism and energy production, plays a significant role in hormone regulation. Thyroid disorders, particularly hypothyroidism (an underactive thyroid), can contribute to low testosterone levels.

Hypothyroidism affects overall endocrine function and can interfere with the body's production and regulation of testosterone.

5. **Chronic Illnesses**

   Chronic illnesses, such as liver or kidney disease, can negatively impact testosterone production. These organs play essential roles in metabolising hormones, and any dysfunction can disrupt the hormonal balance. Men with chronic liver disease, for example, may experience reduced testosterone levels due to the liver's impaired ability to process and eliminate oestrogen, which increases oestrogen levels and reduces testosterone.

6. **Autoimmune Diseases**

   Autoimmune diseases, like rheumatoid arthritis and lupus, can contribute to low testosterone by promoting chronic inflammation in the body. Inflammatory cytokines released by the immune system can suppress testosterone production. Additionally, certain medications used to manage autoimmune conditions may also affect hormone levels.

7. **Cancer and Cancer Treatments**
   Certain cancers, particularly those affecting the testes or pituitary gland, can lead to low testosterone. Cancer treatments, such as chemotherapy and radiation, may damage testosterone-producing cells or disrupt the endocrine system, leading to lower levels. Prostate cancer treatment, specifically androgen deprivation therapy (ADT), is designed to lower testosterone but can lead to long-term deficiency even after treatment concludes.

8. **HIV/AIDS**
   HIV and AIDS can lead to low testosterone due to the virus's effects on the body and immune system. Men with HIV/AIDS often experience hormonal imbalances as the immune system's response affects the endocrine system. Additionally, the medications used to

manage HIV may also lower testosterone levels.

9. **Testicular Injury or Surgery**
Physical damage to the testicles, either from injury or surgery, can directly impact testosterone production. Since the testicles are the primary source of testosterone in men, any significant injury or removal of testicular tissue can lead to permanent declines in testosterone levels.

Testing and Diagnosing Low Testosterone

Low testosterone can lead to a variety of symptoms that affect physical, mental, and emotional well-being. Identifying and diagnosing low testosterone is essential for understanding its impact on health and for developing an effective treatment plan. Testing for testosterone involves a comprehensive approach to understand not just total levels but also the availability and function of testosterone within the body.

When and Why to Get Tested

Recognizing when to test for testosterone is the first step in identifying potential hormone imbalances. Low testosterone, known medically as hypogonadism, is often associated with a set of symptoms that can significantly impact quality of life. Although testosterone naturally declines with age, low levels may sometimes occur earlier or due to underlying health conditions.

1. **Physical Symptoms**
   Physical changes are often the first indicators of low testosterone. Common physical symptoms include reduced muscle mass, increased body fat (especially around the abdomen), decreased bone density, and a decrease in body hair. Men experiencing unexplained fatigue, reduced stamina, or changes in body composition should consider getting tested, especially if these changes are not aligned with ageing or lifestyle factors.

2. **Sexual Health**
   Testosterone plays a key role in male

sexual health, including libido and erectile function. Men who experience a noticeable decrease in sexual desire, difficulties with erectile function, or decreased sexual satisfaction may have low testosterone levels. While these symptoms can have multiple causes, testing testosterone is a helpful first step in identifying potential hormonal causes.

3. **Mood and Mental Health**
   Low testosterone can lead to emotional and psychological changes, such as depression, irritability, difficulty concentrating, and a general lack of motivation. Men experiencing unexplained mood swings or mental fog, particularly alongside physical symptoms, may benefit from a testosterone test to identify possible hormonal influences.

4. **Chronic Health Conditions**
   Men with conditions such as obesity, type 2 diabetes, or metabolic syndrome often have lower testosterone levels due to factors like increased fat tissue, insulin

resistance, and chronic inflammation.
Testing testosterone in these cases can
help with comprehensive management, as
improving testosterone levels may
positively impact overall health.
Additionally, chronic illnesses like
HIV/AIDS, liver disease, and autoimmune
disorders are linked to low testosterone,
and regular testing is often recommended
for those with these conditions.

5. **Age Considerations**
Testosterone levels begin to decline
gradually after age 30. For men over 40,
periodic testing may be beneficial to
monitor how hormone levels are changing
with age. Men over 50 who experience
low-energy, muscle loss, or significant
changes in libido or mood may want to
assess their testosterone to determine if
these issues stem from natural declines or
a more pronounced drop in testosterone.

6. **Pre-Treatment Evaluation**
Before beginning any hormone therapy,
such as testosterone replacement therapy

(TRT), it is essential to establish baseline testosterone levels. Testing provides insight into whether low testosterone is indeed the cause of symptoms and helps to determine the appropriate course of treatment.

Types of Testosterone Tests and What They Measure

Testing for testosterone involves measuring the hormone's levels in the bloodstream. There are different forms of testosterone tests, each providing unique insights into hormone status. The main types of testosterone tests include total testosterone, free testosterone, and bioavailable testosterone.

1. **Total Testosterone Test**
   This test measures the total amount of testosterone in the blood, including both the portion bound to proteins and the unbound (free) portion. Since most testosterone in the blood is bound to sex hormone-binding globulin (SHBG) and

albumin, the total testosterone test gives an overall picture of testosterone levels. However, this measure doesn't always capture how much testosterone is readily available to the body's cells, which is why additional tests are often recommended for more accuracy.

2. **Free Testosterone Test**
Free testosterone refers to the small percentage of testosterone that is not bound to proteins and is freely available to enter cells and carry out its functions. Free testosterone usually makes up about 1-2% of the total testosterone level. This test is particularly useful for assessing the active amount of testosterone available in the bloodstream and can be crucial for diagnosing testosterone deficiency in cases where total testosterone levels are borderline.

3. **Bioavailable Testosterone Test**
Bioavailable testosterone includes free testosterone and testosterone bound to albumin, a protein with a weaker binding

affinity than SHBG. Since albumin-bound testosterone can be easily released and is thus more readily available for use in the body, the bioavailable testosterone test is often a more accurate indicator of functional testosterone levels than total testosterone alone. This test is especially relevant for older men, as SHBG levels tend to increase with age, reducing the amount of free testosterone.

4. **Salivary Testosterone Test**
   While blood tests are the standard for testosterone measurement, salivary testosterone tests offer an alternative method, though they are less widely used in clinical settings. Saliva tests measure free testosterone and can be helpful in assessing diurnal variations in hormone levels. However, due to variability in accuracy, saliva tests are generally considered supplemental rather than primary diagnostic tools.

5. **Additional Hormone Tests**
   A comprehensive evaluation may include

other hormone tests such as LH
(luteinizing hormone), FSH
(follicle-stimulating hormone), and
estradiol (a form of oestrogen). Measuring
LH and FSH can help pinpoint whether
low testosterone is due to primary
hypogonadism (testicular dysfunction) or
secondary hypogonadism (issues with the
pituitary or hypothalamus). Estradiol
testing is important because testosterone
can convert to oestrogen in the body, and
elevated levels may impact symptoms and
treatment choices.

Interpreting Your Testosterone Levels

Interpreting testosterone levels involves more
than simply looking at numbers. Normal ranges
can vary based on age, testing methods, and
individual health conditions. Understanding
what these levels mean requires consideration of
both total testosterone and its active forms, as
well as a context of symptoms and lifestyle.

1. **Reference Ranges**
   Typical reference ranges for testosterone
   vary, but for most adult men, normal total
   testosterone levels are between 300 to
   1,000 ng/dL (nanograms per deciliter).
   Free testosterone levels usually fall
   between 9 to 30 ng/dL. However, these
   ranges are not absolute, and "normal" can
   differ slightly among individuals based on
   factors like age and laboratory standards.

2. **Optimal vs. Normal Levels**
   While a testosterone level may fall within
   the normal range, it may not necessarily
   be optimal for everyone. Some men may
   experience symptoms of low testosterone
   even with levels in the lower part of the
   reference range. Optimal testosterone is
   often individualised and based on where a
   person feels their best, especially if
   symptoms of low testosterone are present
   despite technically normal levels.

3. **Age-Adjusted Levels**
   Since testosterone declines with age,
   levels that are normal for a younger man

may be lower for an older man without causing symptoms. However, if low testosterone is impacting quality of life or contributing to other health issues, treatment options may be explored even if levels are considered age-appropriate.

4. **SHBG and Its Impact on Interpretation**
   Sex hormone-binding globulin (SHBG) is important in interpreting testosterone results, particularly for older men. High SHBG can reduce free testosterone levels, which may lead to symptoms despite normal total testosterone levels. Measuring SHBG alongside testosterone can help in understanding how much testosterone is bioavailable and whether SHBG is impacting testosterone's effectiveness in the body.

5. **Context of Symptoms**
   Testosterone levels should always be interpreted in the context of symptoms. Lab values alone may not fully explain someone's health experience. For example, a man with total testosterone

levels at the lower end of normal but experiencing symptoms like low energy, mood changes, or decreased libido might still benefit from interventions aimed at boosting testosterone.

6. **Follow-Up and Monitoring**

   For those diagnosed with low testosterone, regular follow-up tests can help monitor hormone levels over time. This is especially important for men undergoing testosterone replacement therapy (TRT), as therapy requires careful monitoring to ensure levels remain within a healthy range and to minimise potential side effects. Routine testing every three to six months allows for adjustments in dosage or treatment methods as needed.

Natural Ways to Boost Testosterone

Boosting testosterone levels naturally can have a profound impact on physical health, mental well-being, and overall quality of life. Instead of immediately turning to synthetic supplements or medications, many individuals first explore lifestyle and dietary changes. These natural methods not only help improve testosterone but also contribute to general health and vitality.

Nutrition and Dietary Tips for Optimal Testosterone

Nutrition is a powerful lever when it comes to supporting hormone health, including testosterone production. A well-balanced diet rich in specific nutrients is essential for maintaining optimal testosterone levels, and certain foods can play a pivotal role in supporting the body's natural hormone production.

1. **Consume Healthy Fats**
   Dietary fats are essential for hormone production. Testosterone synthesis depends on cholesterol, so incorporating healthy fats from sources like avocados, olive oil, nuts, seeds, and fatty fish can help ensure the body has the necessary building blocks for testosterone production. Omega-3 fatty acids from fish oil or flaxseeds are particularly beneficial for reducing inflammation and supporting hormonal balance.

2. **Prioritise Protein Intake**
   Protein is crucial for muscle maintenance and repair, which indirectly supports

healthy testosterone levels. Testosterone is heavily involved in muscle growth and repair, so consuming adequate protein helps preserve lean muscle mass, which can positively influence testosterone. Lean meats, poultry, eggs, and legumes are excellent sources of protein that can be part of a balanced diet to support testosterone levels.

3. **Include Zinc-Rich Foods**

   Zinc is one of the most important minerals for testosterone production. Zinc deficiency has been linked to low testosterone levels, and increasing zinc intake can help support the body's natural hormone production. Foods high in zinc include oysters, red meat, pumpkin seeds, and fortified cereals. If dietary intake is insufficient, a high-quality zinc supplement may also be considered after consulting a healthcare provider.

4. **Get Enough Vitamin D**

   Known as the "sunshine vitamin," vitamin D plays a vital role in testosterone production and overall health. Studies have shown that men with adequate vitamin D levels have higher testosterone than those deficient in the vitamin. Regular exposure to sunlight can help boost vitamin D, but supplementation is also an option, especially for individuals who live in areas with limited sun exposure.

5. **Incorporate Magnesium-Rich Foods**
Magnesium helps regulate testosterone by managing oxidative stress and supporting cellular health. This mineral is important for maintaining optimal testosterone levels, particularly for active individuals who may lose magnesium through sweat. Foods rich in magnesium include leafy green vegetables, nuts, seeds, and whole grains.

6. **Limit Processed Foods and Sugars**
Processed foods, particularly those high in sugar and refined carbohydrates, can negatively affect testosterone levels by increasing insulin resistance and

promoting weight gain. Excess body fat can lead to higher oestrogen levels, which can suppress testosterone. Opt for whole, unprocessed foods as often as possible, including fruits, vegetables, lean proteins, and healthy fats to help maintain a balanced hormonal environment.

7. **Moderate Alcohol Intake**
   While moderate alcohol consumption may not significantly impact testosterone, heavy drinking has been shown to lower testosterone levels. Alcohol can disrupt the endocrine system, leading to reduced testosterone production and an increase in cortisol, a stress hormone that negatively affects testosterone. Limiting alcohol intake to moderate levels can help maintain a healthier hormonal balance.

The Role of Exercise in Testosterone Production

Physical activity, particularly strength training and high-intensity interval training (HIIT), has a significant impact on testosterone levels.

Exercise not only promotes the release of testosterone during and after workouts, but it also helps reduce body fat, which is essential for optimising hormone levels.

1. **Strength Training**
   Lifting weights is one of the most effective ways to naturally boost testosterone. Compound movements like squats, deadlifts, bench presses, and rows target multiple muscle groups and stimulate testosterone release. Research shows that resistance training can increase testosterone levels in men, particularly when heavier weights and lower repetitions are used. Training larger muscle groups (e.g., legs and back) also results in a more significant testosterone boost than focusing only on smaller muscles.

2. **High-Intensity Interval Training (HIIT)**
   HIIT involves alternating short bursts of intense activity with periods of rest or low-intensity exercise. This type of

training has been shown to effectively raise testosterone levels while enhancing cardiovascular health and burning fat. HIIT exercises can be tailored to individual fitness levels and can be as simple as sprinting, cycling, or bodyweight exercises done at high intensity. The increase in testosterone from HIIT may also last for hours after the workout, offering prolonged benefits.

3. **Avoid Excessive Endurance Training**
   While moderate aerobic exercise is beneficial for heart health and overall fitness, excessive endurance exercise can have a negative impact on testosterone levels. Long periods of high-endurance training, such as marathon running, can lead to elevated cortisol levels, which can suppress testosterone. For men looking to optimise testosterone, a balance between cardiovascular exercise and resistance training is ideal.

4. **Focus on Recovery**
   Exercise is a form of physical stress, and

recovery is essential for allowing the body to repair, grow, and restore testosterone levels. Overtraining can result in elevated cortisol, which can suppress testosterone production. Ensuring adequate rest between intense workouts, incorporating rest days, and utilising techniques like foam rolling and stretching are crucial for maintaining healthy testosterone levels.

5. **Maintain a Healthy Body Composition** Regular exercise is key to maintaining a healthy weight and reducing excess body fat. Obesity is linked to low testosterone because fat tissue contains an enzyme called aromatase, which converts testosterone to oestrogen. By maintaining a healthy body composition, men can reduce the risk of excess oestrogen, helping testosterone levels remain stable.

Sleep and Stress Management Techniques

Good sleep and stress management are vital for sustaining healthy testosterone levels. Chronic sleep deprivation and high-stress levels can disrupt hormone production, resulting in lower testosterone.

1. **Prioritise Quality Sleep**
   Sleep is one of the most overlooked factors in testosterone production. During deep sleep, the body releases luteinizing hormone (LH), which stimulates testosterone production. Studies show that men who get sufficient, high-quality sleep have higher testosterone levels than those who are sleep-deprived. Aim for 7-8 hours of restful sleep per night, and consider implementing a consistent sleep schedule to support optimal hormone production.

2. **Maintain a Consistent Sleep Schedule**
   Going to bed and waking up at the same time every day, even on weekends, can help regulate the body's circadian rhythm. This consistency supports hormone production, including testosterone. Avoid blue light exposure from screens in the hour leading up to bed, as it can disrupt

melatonin production, which is crucial for a restful night's sleep.

3. **Manage Stress and Cortisol Levels**

   Chronic stress triggers the release of cortisol, a hormone that has a direct inverse relationship with testosterone. When cortisol levels are high, testosterone levels typically decrease. To manage stress, practice relaxation techniques like deep breathing, meditation, yoga, or mindfulness. These practices help to lower cortisol, supporting a better balance of testosterone.

4. **Practise Deep Breathing and Meditation**

   Deep breathing exercises and meditation can significantly reduce stress and improve emotional well-being. These techniques help lower cortisol levels and encourage relaxation, which in turn helps prevent the suppression of testosterone. Even a few minutes of deep breathing or mindfulness practice each day can create a positive impact on stress levels and hormonal balance.

5. **Engage in Relaxing Hobbies and Social Connections**

   Having enjoyable hobbies and positive social connections can help relieve stress and promote mental health. Activities that bring joy or a sense of accomplishment—such as cooking, gardening, or engaging in creative projects—can help manage stress levels. Socialising with family and friends has also been shown to reduce cortisol and support overall well-being, which is beneficial for maintaining healthy testosterone levels.

6. **Limit Stimulants Before Bed**

   Caffeine and other stimulants can interfere with sleep, which indirectly impacts testosterone production. Avoid consuming caffeine in the afternoon or evening to support a good night's sleep. Instead, consider calming teas like chamomile or valerian root, which may help relax the body and improve sleep quality.

Testosterone and Sexual Health

Testosterone is often referred to as the "male sex hormone" because of its critical role in sexual health and function. This powerful hormone affects libido, sexual performance, erectile function, and overall satisfaction with one's intimate life. Both men and women produce testosterone, though in different amounts, and it serves as a crucial component for various aspects of reproductive health.

Testosterone's Role in Libido and Sexual Performance

Libido, or sexual drive, is influenced by several factors, with testosterone being one of the most important. Testosterone acts on specific brain regions to stimulate the desire for sexual activity, creating a strong connection between testosterone levels and libido.

1. **Testosterone as a Driver of Sexual Desire**

   Testosterone impacts the hypothalamus in the brain, an area involved in regulating sexual drive and arousal. When testosterone levels are adequate, it signals the brain to increase interest and responsiveness to sexual cues, boosting sexual desire and motivation. Low levels of testosterone, however, can reduce these signals, leading to a noticeable drop in libido. For men, this drop can be gradual with age, but in some cases, factors like stress, obesity, or underlying health issues can lead to early declines in testosterone, impacting sexual desire prematurely.

2. **Testosterone's Role in Energy and Stamina**

   Testosterone plays a role in physical energy and stamina, which are essential for sexual performance. This hormone aids in protein synthesis and muscle strength, which help maintain physical endurance and resilience. Low testosterone can result in fatigue and decreased physical strength, impacting sexual performance and contributing to a lower sex drive.

3. **Mood and Confidence**
   Testosterone also affects mood and confidence, both of which are indirectly linked to sexual health. Lower testosterone levels can contribute to feelings of depression, low self-esteem, and reduced confidence, all of which can diminish sexual interest and satisfaction. Men and women who experience low testosterone may feel less inclined toward intimacy or might experience performance anxiety, further impacting their sexual relationships.

4. **Impact on Sexual Responsiveness**
   Research indicates that testosterone not only affects the desire for sex but also

physical responsiveness. In men, testosterone is linked to physical sensitivity in the erogenous zones, meaning that low testosterone levels can impact the physical response to sexual stimuli, reducing the sensation and pleasure experienced during intimacy. In women, testosterone influences both the libido and aspects of sensitivity, contributing to overall sexual satisfaction.

Erectile Function and Testosterone Levels

Erectile function is a complex physiological process that involves a delicate balance of blood flow, nervous system responses, and hormonal regulation. Testosterone is crucial for erectile health and affects it in a few key ways.

1. **Testosterone's Role in Nitric Oxide Production**
   Testosterone helps stimulate the production of nitric oxide, a molecule that plays a significant role in erectile function. Nitric oxide facilitates the

relaxation of blood vessels, allowing blood to flow into the penile tissues, which is necessary for achieving and maintaining an erection. When testosterone levels are low, nitric oxide production can also decrease, which may result in poor blood flow and lead to erectile dysfunction (ED).

2. **Influence on Penile Tissue and Receptors**

   Testosterone also affects the tissues within the penis. Studies show that low testosterone can lead to reduced elasticity in the penile tissue, which is necessary for achieving a firm erection. Additionally, testosterone interacts with receptors in the penile tissue that facilitate smooth muscle relaxation during arousal, which is essential for maintaining an erection.

3. **Hormonal Balance and Erectile Dysfunction**

   Testosterone is not the sole factor involved in erectile function, but it plays a foundational role. Other hormones, such as dopamine, prolactin, and oxytocin, also influence sexual health, but testosterone is essential for maintaining an optimal hormonal environment for erections. When testosterone levels are low, these hormones can become imbalanced, leading to issues with arousal, erectile strength, and duration.

4. **Psychological Aspect of Erectile Function**

Erectile dysfunction can have a psychological component as well. Testosterone helps maintain mental sharpness, focus, and confidence, all of which contribute to sexual function. Men with low testosterone often report higher levels of performance anxiety, reduced confidence in their abilities, and stress over sexual encounters. By addressing low testosterone, many men can alleviate some of the psychological burdens that affect erectile performance.

Common Sexual Health Issues Linked to Testosterone

Low testosterone levels can be linked to a range of sexual health issues, affecting both men and women. While men experience more direct impacts on erectile function and libido, women may also suffer from decreased sexual desire and satisfaction. Here are some common sexual health concerns related to testosterone levels:

1. **Low Libido**

    One of the most common symptoms of low testosterone is a decreased sex drive. In men, a noticeable drop in sexual interest is often one of the first signs of low testosterone, particularly if it happens suddenly or in early adulthood. For women, low testosterone can also decrease libido, though it may be less noticeable since women typically have lower baseline levels of testosterone. Reversing low testosterone levels can help restore libido in both men and women.

2. **Erectile Dysfunction**

   Erectile dysfunction is a multifaceted condition influenced by physical, hormonal, and psychological factors. Testosterone's role in nitric oxide production and blood flow regulation means that low testosterone can directly contribute to erectile dysfunction. Low testosterone levels do not necessarily cause ED alone, but they can exacerbate the condition, particularly in men who are already dealing with vascular or nervous system issues.

3. **Reduced Sexual Satisfaction**

   Beyond libido and erectile function, low testosterone can also impact overall satisfaction with sexual experiences. Low levels of testosterone may lead to a decrease in pleasure, sensitivity, and satisfaction during sexual activity. For men, this may manifest as a lack of physical response to arousal, while for women, it can lead to decreased arousal and reduced sensitivity, affecting the overall sexual experience.

4. **Fatigue and Lack of Stamina**
Fatigue is a common symptom of low testosterone and can significantly impact sexual activity. Men with low testosterone often report feeling too tired to engage in sexual activity or experiencing fatigue that prevents them from enjoying the experience fully. Addressing testosterone deficiencies can often improve energy levels, helping individuals feel more motivated and engaged in intimate relationships.

5. **Mood-Related Sexual Issues**
Low testosterone can affect mood, leading to irritability, depression, and anxiety. These mood changes can have a profound impact on sexual health, as stress and negative emotions can create a barrier to intimacy. Depression, in particular, is known to reduce libido, while anxiety can lead to performance concerns in men. Restoring testosterone levels may help

improve mood stability, thereby enhancing overall sexual satisfaction.

6. **Difficulty Achieving Orgasm**
   Both men and women with low testosterone may experience difficulty achieving orgasm. Testosterone influences the brain's sexual response, affecting the intensity and duration of pleasure. Low levels can make it challenging for individuals to reach orgasm, which can contribute to a lack of fulfilment and satisfaction in their sexual experiences.

Medical Treatments for Low Testosterone

Medical treatments for low testosterone have become more refined and accessible, allowing individuals with testosterone deficiencies to regain a healthier hormonal balance. One of the most widely used treatments is Testosterone Replacement Therapy (TRT), which is specifically designed to restore testosterone to optimal levels. TRT can provide a range of benefits, including improved mood, increased energy, enhanced libido, and better overall well-being. However, understanding the various forms of TRT and the potential risks and benefits is crucial before beginning any hormone replacement regimen.

Overview of Testosterone Replacement Therapy (TRT)

Testosterone Replacement Therapy (TRT) involves supplementing the body's natural testosterone levels to counteract the symptoms of testosterone deficiency. For many men, TRT is a lifeline that restores energy, mood, libido, and physical strength that may have been diminished due to low testosterone. Though TRT is most commonly associated with men, women with low testosterone can also benefit from hormone therapy, though typically at much lower doses.

1. **How TRT Works**
   TRT works by introducing synthetic testosterone into the body to compensate for what the body no longer produces sufficiently. This therapy can help alleviate symptoms such as fatigue, depression, low libido, and muscle loss.

While it doesn't cure the underlying cause of low testosterone, TRT can effectively manage the symptoms associated with the condition.

2. **Who Can Benefit from TRT**
   TRT is generally recommended for individuals with clinically low testosterone levels, which are confirmed through blood tests. TRT may be particularly beneficial for men over the age of 40 who experience age-related testosterone decline or individuals who have testosterone deficiency due to medical conditions, such as hypogonadism or chronic illnesses. Before beginning TRT, patients undergo a thorough evaluation, including hormone testing and an assessment of medical history to determine if they are a suitable candidate.

3. **Primary Goals of TRT**
   The primary objective of TRT is to restore testosterone levels within the normal physiological range, relieving symptoms

associated with low testosterone and improving the quality of life. Secondary goals often include enhancing mood, restoring sexual function, and supporting muscle growth and bone density. TRT is not typically recommended solely for enhancing athletic performance or for anti-aging purposes unless low testosterone is clinically indicated.

Different Forms of TRT: Injections, Patches, and Gels

TRT comes in several forms, allowing patients to choose an option that best suits their lifestyle, medical needs, and preferences. The main delivery methods include injections, transdermal patches, and topical gels. Each method has its unique advantages and considerations.

1. **Injections**
   Testosterone injections are among the most common and effective forms of TRT. The injections deliver a specific dose of testosterone directly into the bloodstream,

providing a rapid and noticeable increase in testosterone levels. Injections are usually administered in a medical setting, though some patients may self-inject at home under the guidance of a healthcare provider.

- **Types of Injections**: There are short-acting and long-acting injections available. Short-acting injections, such as testosterone cypionate or enanthate, are typically administered every 1-2 weeks, while long-acting versions, such as testosterone undecanoate, may only need to be administered every 10-12 weeks.
- **Advantages**: Injections allow for controlled dosing and immediate testosterone elevation. For many, they are cost-effective and convenient in terms of frequency.
- **Considerations**: Some patients may experience fluctuations in testosterone levels between

injections, leading to "highs" and "lows" in energy and mood. Additionally, injections can sometimes cause discomfort at the injection site and require regular administration.

2. **Patches**

Testosterone patches are applied to the skin and deliver a steady dose of testosterone through the bloodstream over 24 hours. They are typically worn on the back, thighs, abdomen, or upper arms.

- **Advantages**: Patches provide a consistent release of testosterone, avoiding the peaks and valleys that can occur with injections. This method may feel more natural and is less invasive than injections.

- **Considerations**: Some patients find patches uncomfortable, as they may cause skin irritation or rashes at the application site. The patches must be changed daily, which can be inconvenient for some.

Additionally, this form of TRT may be less effective for individuals with high levels of physical activity, as sweating can reduce patch adherence.

3. **Gels and Creams**

   Testosterone gels and creams are applied topically to areas such as the shoulders, arms, or abdomen, where they are absorbed through the skin. Gels are typically applied daily and can provide consistent testosterone levels similar to patches.

   - **Advantages**: Gels and creams are non-invasive and can be applied at home. They offer a more consistent delivery method than injections and are generally easy to use.
   - **Considerations**: One of the primary concerns with gels and creams is the risk of transferring testosterone to others through skin contact. Patients must avoid direct contact with others, especially

children and women, until the gel
has dried. Daily application can
also be a disadvantage for those
who prefer less frequent dosing.

4. **Pellets**

Less commonly, testosterone pellets are a
form of TRT that involves implanting
small pellets under the skin, usually in the
buttocks or hip area. These pellets
gradually release testosterone over a few
months.

- **Advantages**: Pellets provide a
  long-lasting effect, requiring
  minimal maintenance and avoiding
  daily or weekly applications. The
  hormone is absorbed slowly and
  steadily, leading to more stable
  testosterone levels.
- **Considerations**: Pellet insertion
  requires a minor surgical procedure
  and can cause discomfort.
  Additionally, pellets may
  occasionally work their way out of
  the skin, requiring replacement.

Potential Risks and Benefits of Testosterone Therapy

While TRT can provide significant benefits, it also comes with potential risks. Understanding both the benefits and risks helps patients make informed decisions about starting or continuing testosterone therapy.

1. **Benefits of Testosterone Therapy**
   TRT can offer substantial health and lifestyle benefits for those experiencing low testosterone. Some of the primary benefits include:
     - **Improved Sexual Health**: One of the most immediate benefits of TRT is its impact on sexual health. Testosterone therapy can help restore libido, improve erectile function, and enhance sexual satisfaction for those suffering from low testosterone.
     - **Enhanced Mood and Cognitive Function**: Low testosterone is linked to symptoms like depression,

irritability, and cognitive fog. Many patients report improved mood stability, sharper focus, and better mental clarity with TRT.

- o **Increased Muscle Mass and Bone Density**: Testosterone plays a crucial role in muscle growth and bone health. TRT can help those with low testosterone improve muscle mass and strength, reducing the risk of falls and fractures in older men.
- o **Higher Energy Levels**: Fatigue and low energy are common symptoms of testosterone deficiency. By restoring testosterone levels, TRT can help individuals feel more energised and motivated, improving overall quality of life.

2. **Potential Risks and Side Effects of Testosterone Therapy**

Although beneficial, TRT is not without

its risks and side effects. Some potential risks of TRT include:

- **Cardiovascular Issues**: Some studies suggest a link between TRT and an increased risk of heart disease, though this association remains under debate. Men with pre-existing heart conditions should discuss TRT carefully with their healthcare provider.

- **Increased Red Blood Cell Count**: Testosterone therapy can raise red blood cell levels, which may increase the risk of blood clots and related complications, such as deep vein thrombosis or stroke.

- **Prostate Health Concerns**: While TRT does not directly cause prostate cancer, it can stimulate growth in the prostate, potentially exacerbating benign prostatic hyperplasia (BPH) or contributing to prostate health concerns.

- ○ **Hormonal Imbalances**:
  Introducing synthetic testosterone can disrupt the natural balance of hormones, leading to issues such as testicular shrinkage, infertility, and a decrease in natural testosterone production.

3. **Considering the Long-Term Implications**

Testosterone therapy requires long-term commitment, and ceasing TRT can lead to a rapid decline in testosterone levels. For some individuals, TRT may require lifelong treatment to maintain hormone balance, especially if the underlying cause of low testosterone is age-related. Regular follow-up with a healthcare provider, including monitoring of hormone levels, prostate health, and cardiovascular risk factors, is essential to mitigate potential risks.

The Role of Supplements in Testosterone Health

In addition to lifestyle changes, dietary improvements, and medical treatments, supplements have gained popularity as a natural way to support healthy testosterone levels. With the rise of fitness and wellness culture, many individuals are looking for ways to boost their testosterone levels without resorting to prescription treatments like Testosterone Replacement Therapy (TRT). Supplements marketed as testosterone boosters can play a role in maintaining or even increasing testosterone production, especially when paired with a healthy diet and exercise regimen. However, while some supplements show promise, others lack sufficient evidence to support their claims.

Common Supplements for Supporting Testosterone

A variety of supplements claim to help raise or maintain testosterone levels. These include vitamins, minerals, herbs, amino acids, and other natural compounds. While the effectiveness of these supplements may vary, many have been studied for their potential to support testosterone health. Below are some of the most common supplements used to support testosterone levels:

1. **Vitamin D**

   Vitamin D is a crucial nutrient for overall health, and research suggests that it may play a role in testosterone production. Studies have shown that men with low levels of vitamin D are more likely to have low testosterone levels, and supplementation with vitamin D can help raise both total and free testosterone levels in some individuals.

- **How It Works**: Vitamin D acts on the endocrine system by enhancing the secretion of luteinizing hormone (LH), which in turn stimulates testosterone production. It also has anti-inflammatory properties that can contribute to overall hormonal balance.
- **Recommended Dosage**: The typical recommended dosage ranges from 1,000 to 5,000 IU per day, depending on individual needs and blood test results.

2. **Zinc**

Zinc is an essential mineral that plays a vital role in testosterone synthesis. Zinc deficiency has been linked to reduced testosterone levels, and supplementation can help boost testosterone levels in zinc-deficient individuals.

- ○ **How It Works**: Zinc supports the production of both luteinizing hormone and testosterone. It also has antioxidant properties that protect against oxidative stress, which can negatively impact testosterone levels.
- ○ **Recommended Dosage**: The recommended daily intake of zinc for men is about 11 mg, though supplementation doses can range from 15 to 30 mg per day.

3. **Magnesium**

Magnesium is another mineral that supports testosterone health. Like zinc, magnesium deficiency has been linked to lower testosterone levels. Supplementing with magnesium may help improve testosterone production, especially in men who are deficient in this mineral.

- ○ **How It Works**: Magnesium helps regulate testosterone by enhancing the actions of certain enzymes involved in testosterone production.

It also supports the body's ability to manage stress, which can otherwise contribute to lowered testosterone levels.

- ○ **Recommended Dosage**: A typical magnesium supplement dose ranges from 200 to 400 mg per day, depending on individual needs.

4. **Ashwagandha**

Ashwagandha, an adaptogenic herb used in traditional Ayurvedic medicine, has become a popular supplement for testosterone health. Studies suggest that ashwagandha may help boost testosterone levels, particularly in men experiencing high levels of stress or who are undergoing physical training.

- ○ **How It Works**: Ashwagandha has been shown to reduce cortisol levels (a stress hormone) and increase luteinizing hormone, which can stimulate testosterone production. It also helps reduce inflammation and improve overall vitality.

- o **Recommended Dosage**: Ashwagandha is typically taken in doses of 300 to 500 mg per day of an extract standardised to contain 5% withanolides.

5. **Fenugreek**

Fenugreek is a herb that has been traditionally used to support male health. Research indicates that fenugreek supplementation may improve testosterone levels, particularly in individuals with low testosterone or those undergoing intense exercise.

- o **How It Works**: Fenugreek contains compounds called saponins, which are thought to enhance testosterone production by promoting the release of luteinizing hormone and by inhibiting the enzyme aromatase, which converts testosterone into oestrogen.
- o **Recommended Dosage**: Typical doses of fenugreek extract range from 500 to 600 mg per day.

6. **D-Aspartic Acid**

   D-Aspartic acid is an amino acid that plays a key role in the synthesis of testosterone. Research suggests that this amino acid may increase testosterone levels in certain individuals, particularly those who are infertile or have low testosterone.

   - **How It Works**: D-Aspartic acid works by stimulating the production of luteinizing hormone, which in turn triggers the Leydig cells in the testes to produce testosterone.
   - **Recommended Dosage**: D-Aspartic acid is typically taken in doses of 2,000 to 3,000 mg per day.

7. **Tribulus Terrestris**

   Tribulus Terrestris is a plant extract commonly used in traditional medicine to support male reproductive health. While its effectiveness in boosting testosterone is debated, some studies suggest that it may help improve sexual health and vitality.

- ○ **How It Works**: Tribulus may influence testosterone levels by boosting levels of certain hormones, including luteinizing hormone. However, its effect on testosterone production may be mild compared to other supplements.
- ○ **Recommended Dosage**: Typical doses of Tribulus Terrestris range from 250 to 1,500 mg per day, depending on the concentration of active ingredients.

Pros and Cons of Testosterone-Boosting Supplements

While many testosterone-boosting supplements show promise, there are both benefits and limitations to consider before incorporating them into your health regimen.

Pros:

- **Non-invasive and Easy to Use:** Supplements offer a convenient way to support testosterone levels without the need for injections or prescriptions.

- **Natural Ingredients**: Many testosterone-boosting supplements contain natural ingredients like herbs and vitamins, which may be more appealing to those seeking holistic or natural health solutions.

- **Improved Well-being**: For individuals with nutrient deficiencies, supplements like vitamin D, zinc, and magnesium may help improve not only testosterone levels but also overall health, including immune function, mood, and energy.

- **Support for Lifestyle Changes**: When combined with proper exercise, diet, and sleep, supplements can enhance the effects of lifestyle changes aimed at optimising testosterone levels.

Cons:

- **Limited Scientific Evidence**: While many testosterone-boosting supplements are popular, scientific evidence supporting their effectiveness is often limited. The impact of these supplements can vary significantly between individuals, and the effects may not be as profound as some claims suggest.

- **Possible Side Effects**: Some supplements can cause adverse effects, such as digestive issues, skin reactions, or hormonal imbalances. For example, excessive zinc intake can lead to copper deficiency, and high doses of magnesium can cause diarrhoea.

- **No Substitute for Medical Treatment**: Supplements are not a replacement for medical therapies, especially for individuals with clinically low testosterone due to medical conditions. While supplements can help support healthy testosterone levels, they may not be sufficient for treating severe testosterone deficiencies.

Safety and Effectiveness of Natural Alternatives

When considering natural alternatives for boosting testosterone, it is important to approach supplements with caution. Here are several key considerations for ensuring safety and effectiveness:

1. **Consulting a Healthcare Provider**: Before starting any supplementation regimen, it's crucial to consult with a healthcare provider. They can recommend appropriate doses, check for nutrient deficiencies, and monitor progress. This is especially important for individuals with underlying health conditions like heart disease or prostate issues.
2. **Quality and Purity**: Not all supplements are created equal. Some testosterone-boosting supplements may contain contaminants or suboptimal doses of active ingredients. Look for products that are third-party tested and certified for purity.
3. **Holistic Approach**: Supplements are most effective when combined with a

healthy lifestyle. Prioritise exercise, good nutrition, adequate sleep, and stress management to optimise testosterone production naturally.

4. **Be Sceptical of Overly Bold Claims**: Many testosterone supplements are marketed with exaggerated claims, promising dramatic results. While some of these supplements may have a mild impact, they are unlikely to produce the extreme effects often suggested in advertisements.

Testosterone and Aging

As men age, testosterone levels naturally decline, a process that typically begins after the age of 30. This gradual reduction in testosterone can have significant effects on a man's physical, mental, and emotional well-being. Understanding how testosterone functions as we age, the potential impact of low testosterone, and ways to manage these changes is critical for maintaining optimal health throughout the ageing process.

Managing Testosterone Levels as You Age

The decline in testosterone levels with age is a normal part of the ageing process, but the rate at which it declines and its impact can vary significantly from person to person. For some men, testosterone levels may drop at a gradual and relatively benign pace, while for others, it may be more pronounced and lead to noticeable symptoms.

- **Gradual Decline**: Testosterone levels typically begin to decline at a rate of about 1% per year starting in a man's early 30s. By the time they reach their 40s or 50s, some men may start to experience the symptoms associated with lower testosterone levels.
- **Symptoms of Age-Related Testosterone Decline**: These symptoms include fatigue, decreased libido, reduced muscle mass and strength, increased body fat, decreased bone density, irritability, and difficulties with concentration and memory. These changes can contribute to a reduced quality of life and a general sense of ageing or "slowing down."
- **Testosterone Replacement Therapy (TRT)**: For some older men experiencing

significant symptoms of low testosterone, testosterone replacement therapy (TRT) can be an option. TRT aims to bring testosterone levels back to a more youthful range, potentially improving symptoms such as low energy, sexual dysfunction, and decreased muscle mass. However, the decision to undergo TRT should be made in consultation with a healthcare provider, as there are potential risks and benefits to consider.

Benefits and Risks of TRT for Older Adults

Testosterone replacement therapy can provide significant benefits for some older adults, but it is not without its risks. The decision to pursue TRT should be made carefully, weighing the potential rewards against the possible complications.

Benefits of TRT for Older Adults

1. **Improved Energy Levels and Mood**: One of the most noticeable benefits of

TRT is an increase in energy levels. Many men report feeling more energetic, less fatigued, and more motivated after beginning testosterone therapy. Additionally, TRT can have a positive effect on mood, reducing feelings of irritability or depression that can accompany low testosterone.

2. **Enhanced Sexual Function**: Testosterone plays a crucial role in sexual health, and low levels can lead to reduced libido, erectile dysfunction, and other sexual issues. TRT can help restore sexual desire and improve erectile function in some men, leading to a more satisfying sexual experience.

3. **Increased Muscle Mass and Strength**: Testosterone is essential for muscle growth and maintenance. As testosterone levels decline with age, muscle mass tends to decrease, and body fat may increase. By restoring testosterone levels through TRT, some men experience an increase in muscle mass and strength, which can

improve overall physical function and mobility.

4. **Bone Health**: Testosterone has a direct impact on bone density. Low testosterone levels are associated with an increased risk of osteoporosis, making bones more fragile and prone to fractures. TRT can help maintain or increase bone density, reducing the risk of osteoporosis and fractures in older men.

5. **Cognitive Function**: Testosterone has been linked to cognitive functions such as memory, focus, and spatial ability. Some studies suggest that TRT may help with cognitive function in men with low testosterone, though research in this area is still ongoing.

Risks of TRT for Older Adults

1. **Cardiovascular Risks**: One of the most concerning potential risks of TRT for older men is its effect on cardiovascular health. Some studies have suggested that TRT may increase the risk of heart attack,

stroke, and other cardiovascular events, particularly in men who already have underlying heart conditions. It is essential to undergo a thorough cardiovascular evaluation before starting TRT.

2. **Prostate Health**: Testosterone is known to stimulate the growth of prostate tissue, which raises concerns about the potential risk of prostate cancer. Although the link between TRT and prostate cancer remains debated, men with a history of prostate cancer or elevated prostate-specific antigen (PSA) levels should approach TRT with caution. Regular monitoring of PSA levels and prostate health is essential for men undergoing testosterone therapy.

3. **Sleep Apnea**: TRT has been associated with an increased risk of sleep apnea, a condition in which breathing temporarily stops during sleep. This is particularly concerning for older men who may already have an increased risk of sleep-related breathing issues. Men with a history of sleep apnea or breathing

problems should discuss the potential risks of TRT with their healthcare provider.

4. **Blood Clots and Hematocrit Levels**: TRT may increase red blood cell production, which can lead to higher hematocrit levels (the percentage of red blood cells in the blood). This can increase the risk of blood clots, potentially leading to deep vein thrombosis (DVT) or pulmonary embolism. Regular monitoring of hematocrit levels is necessary for men on TRT.

5. **Fertility Concerns**: For men who wish to maintain fertility, TRT may not be an ideal solution. Testosterone therapy can suppress sperm production, potentially leading to infertility. Men who are considering fathering children should discuss this with their healthcare provider and explore alternative treatments.

Healthy Aging Tips for Optimal Hormone Balance

While testosterone replacement therapy may be a beneficial option for some older adults, it is not the only way to maintain healthy testosterone levels as you age. Several lifestyle changes can support the body's natural testosterone production and promote overall hormone balance for healthy ageing. Here are some key tips for maintaining optimal testosterone levels as you age:

1. **Maintain a Healthy Diet**:
   A balanced diet rich in vitamins, minerals, healthy fats, and lean protein is essential for hormone health. Key nutrients that support testosterone production include vitamin D, zinc, magnesium, and healthy fats (such as those found in avocados, olive oil, and fatty fish). Avoid excessive sugar, refined carbohydrates, and processed foods, which can negatively impact hormone levels and lead to inflammation.

2. **Exercise Regularly**:
   Regular physical activity, particularly

resistance training and high-intensity interval training (HIIT), has been shown to increase testosterone levels. Strength training exercises, such as weightlifting, stimulate muscle growth, which in turn boosts testosterone production. Cardiovascular exercise also helps maintain a healthy weight and reduces fat, which can have a positive impact on testosterone levels.

3. **Prioritise Sleep**:
Testosterone production is closely tied to sleep quality. Men who do not get enough sleep (7-9 hours per night) or experience poor-quality sleep may have lower testosterone levels. Aim for a consistent sleep schedule, create a relaxing bedtime routine, and ensure your sleep environment is conducive to restfulness (e.g., keeping the room cool, dark, and quiet).

4. **Manage Stress**:
Chronic stress leads to elevated cortisol levels, which can suppress testosterone

production. Managing stress through relaxation techniques such as meditation, yoga, deep breathing exercises, or mindfulness can help regulate cortisol levels and support hormone balance. Taking time for hobbies, spending time with loved ones, and practising self-care are also important for reducing stress.

5. **Maintain a Healthy Weight**: Excess body fat, particularly abdominal fat, is associated with lower testosterone levels. Maintaining a healthy weight through proper diet and exercise can help optimise testosterone production. Avoiding obesity and keeping your body fat percentage within a healthy range is one of the most important factors for supporting testosterone levels as you age.

6. **Avoid Excessive Alcohol and Smoking**: Both alcohol and smoking can negatively affect testosterone levels. Excessive alcohol consumption can reduce testosterone production, while smoking increases the risk of erectile dysfunction

and other sexual health problems.
Reducing or eliminating these habits can
have a positive impact on your hormone
health and overall well-being.

7. **Regular Health Check-ups**:
Regular medical check-ups are essential
for monitoring testosterone levels and
overall health as you age. Routine blood
tests can help detect any underlying health
conditions, such as thyroid disorders,
diabetes, or sleep apnea, that may impact
testosterone levels. Early detection of any
issues allows for timely intervention and
management.

Testosterone, Mood, and Mental Health

Testosterone is widely known for its role in physical health, influencing muscle mass, bone density, and sexual function. However, its impact extends far beyond just physical traits. Testosterone also plays a critical role in mental health, influencing mood, cognitive function, and emotional well-being. As testosterone levels fluctuate, particularly in men, the effects on mental health can be profound. Understanding how testosterone interacts with mood and emotions, recognizing the signs of low testosterone-related mental health issues, and exploring treatment options are essential for managing overall well-being.

How Testosterone Influences Mood and Emotional Health

Testosterone is a powerful hormone that affects many aspects of physical and mental health. While it is primarily known for its role in muscle growth, libido, and reproductive health, testosterone also directly influences brain function and mood regulation.

1. **Mood Regulation**:
   Testosterone levels have a direct impact on neurotransmitters in the brain, particularly those associated with mood regulation, such as serotonin and dopamine. These neurotransmitters are responsible for feelings of happiness, pleasure, and overall emotional well-being. Testosterone helps to balance these chemicals, promoting a more stable and positive mood. Low testosterone levels can disrupt this balance, potentially

leading to irritability, sadness, and mood
swings.

2. **Confidence and Motivation**:
Testosterone also contributes to feelings
of confidence and motivation, as it
influences areas of the brain that regulate
self-esteem and goal-directed behaviour.
Men with optimal testosterone levels tend
to feel more driven, confident, and
focused on achieving their goals.
Conversely, low testosterone can lead to a
lack of initiative, diminished self-esteem,
and a sense of apathy.

3. **Aggression and Irritability**:
Testosterone has been linked to increased
aggression in some individuals. However,
this aggression is often misunderstood.
While testosterone can increase feelings
of competitiveness and assertiveness, it
can also contribute to irritability or a low
tolerance for frustration, especially when
levels are either too low or imbalanced.
This can lead to sudden outbursts of anger
or frustration, negatively affecting

personal relationships and mental well-being.

4. **Cognitive Function and Clarity**:
Testosterone levels also affect cognitive function, including memory, attention, and mental clarity. Adequate testosterone levels support optimal brain function, helping individuals to think clearly, retain information, and stay mentally sharp. As testosterone levels decline, particularly with age, men may experience cognitive difficulties, such as forgetfulness, lack of focus, and reduced mental agility, which can contribute to a decline in overall mood and well-being.

5. **Stress Response**:
Testosterone has an important role in how the body responds to stress. Low testosterone levels can amplify the body's stress response, increasing cortisol levels, which in turn can exacerbate feelings of anxiety and depression. The imbalance of cortisol, the stress hormone, and testosterone can create a cycle of chronic

stress and emotional instability, further affecting mental health.

Recognizing Symptoms of Low Testosterone Depression

When testosterone levels drop, one of the most common consequences is a shift in mood, which can often resemble or trigger depressive symptoms. Recognizing the signs of low testosterone-induced depression is crucial for proper diagnosis and treatment.

1. **Fatigue and Lack of Energy**:
   One of the hallmark symptoms of low testosterone is overwhelming fatigue, even after adequate rest. Men with low testosterone often report feeling exhausted and lacking energy for both physical activities and everyday tasks. This sense of tiredness can extend to mental energy, causing feelings of mental fog, lack of motivation, and emotional numbness.
2. **Depressed Mood**:
   Low testosterone is closely linked to

depression, and many individuals with low testosterone experience persistent feelings of sadness or hopelessness. The emotional state of sadness often stems from the loss of motivation, reduced energy, and the inability to find joy in activities that once provided pleasure. These feelings are not just situational but can become chronic when testosterone levels remain low over time.

3. **Irritability and Mood Swings**: Irritability is another common symptom of low testosterone. Men may find themselves feeling unusually angry or frustrated over small triggers or situations. This emotional volatility can lead to mood swings, where a person may feel intense anger one moment and then experience sadness or apathy shortly after. The sudden changes in emotional states can strain relationships and affect one's overall sense of emotional stability.

4. **Decreased Libido and Sexual Disinterest**:

Testosterone plays a crucial role in regulating sexual desire. As testosterone levels decline, so does libido. This reduction in sexual interest can contribute to feelings of inadequacy, frustration, and low self-esteem. For many men, a decreased desire for sex is not just a physical symptom but an emotional one as well, leading to feelings of depression and emotional withdrawal.

5. **Cognitive Decline**:
   Testosterone's influence on cognitive function means that men with low testosterone may also experience issues with concentration, memory, and mental clarity. These cognitive impairments can lead to frustration and a sense of helplessness, especially if they interfere with daily activities, work, or social interactions. Cognitive decline often exacerbates feelings of depression, as individuals may become more aware of their mental and emotional struggles.

6. **Sleep Disturbances**:
   Testosterone has a direct connection to the sleep cycle. Low testosterone can lead to sleep disturbances such as insomnia or fragmented sleep, which in turn can worsen symptoms of depression. Poor sleep quality can have a profound impact on mood, making it more difficult to manage emotional health and exacerbating feelings of fatigue and irritability.

7. **Loss of Self-Esteem and Motivation**:
   As testosterone declines, men may experience a decrease in self-esteem and a lack of drive. Low testosterone can cause feelings of inadequacy or a lack of control over one's life. Individuals may no longer feel capable of achieving their goals or taking pride in their accomplishments. This loss of self-worth is a common manifestation of low testosterone-induced depression.

Treatment Options for Mood and Mental Health

When low testosterone is identified as a contributing factor to depression or emotional instability, there are several treatment options available to improve mood and overall mental health. These treatments aim to restore testosterone to optimal levels and address the symptoms of depression and other emotional issues that may arise.

1. **Testosterone Replacement Therapy (TRT):**
   The most direct treatment for low testosterone is testosterone replacement therapy (TRT). This treatment involves supplementing the body with synthetic testosterone through various forms, including injections, gels, patches, or pellets. By restoring testosterone levels, TRT can help alleviate the mood disturbances, fatigue, and irritability associated with low testosterone, potentially improving overall mental health.
   While TRT can significantly improve

mood and mental well-being, it is not a quick fix. It may take several weeks or even months for individuals to notice substantial changes in their emotional state and energy levels. Furthermore, TRT should be carefully monitored by a healthcare provider to ensure that testosterone levels are in the optimal range and that there are no adverse side effects.

2. **Cognitive Behavioral Therapy (CBT):** For men experiencing low testosterone-related depression, cognitive behavioural therapy (CBT) can be an effective adjunct treatment. CBT helps individuals identify negative thought patterns and replace them with healthier, more positive perspectives. It can be particularly useful for addressing the emotional and psychological symptoms of depression, such as low self-esteem, irritability, and apathy.

   In conjunction with hormone therapy, CBT can provide individuals with coping strategies to manage emotional ups and downs and improve overall mental health. This therapy is also beneficial for addressing any underlying anxiety or mood disorders that may be exacerbated by hormonal imbalances.

3. **Lifestyle Modifications**:
Healthy lifestyle changes can also play a significant role in managing the mood and mental health symptoms associated with low testosterone. Regular exercise, especially strength training, can stimulate the natural production of testosterone and improve mood. Exercise increases the release of endorphins, which help reduce feelings of stress, anxiety, and depression. Additionally, dietary changes such as incorporating nutrient-rich foods that support hormone health (like vitamin D, zinc, and healthy fats) can promote balanced testosterone levels. Proper sleep hygiene and stress management techniques, including mindfulness, meditation, or yoga, can also reduce the

psychological effects of low testosterone and support mental well-being.

4. **Medications for Depression**:
   In cases where depression persists despite efforts to address the underlying hormonal imbalance, medications such as antidepressants (SSRIs or SNRIs) may be prescribed to help alleviate depressive symptoms. These medications work by balancing neurotransmitter levels in the brain, helping to improve mood and emotional stability.

5. **Support Groups and Counseling**:
   Emotional support plays a vital role in managing low testosterone and related mental health issues. Support groups for men experiencing similar symptoms can provide a sense of community and help reduce feelings of isolation. Additionally, talking to a mental health professional who specialises in hormonal imbalances can help individuals understand how testosterone levels affect mood and provide coping strategies.

Lifestyle Adjustments for Lasting Testosterone Health

Maintaining healthy testosterone levels is vital for overall well-being, and making the right lifestyle adjustments can have a profound impact on both your physical and mental health. Rather than relying solely on medication or supplements, adopting a testosterone-friendly lifestyle provides a natural, sustainable approach to supporting hormonal balance.

Creating a Testosterone-Friendly Lifestyle

A testosterone-friendly lifestyle isn't just about following quick fixes or jumping on the latest wellness trends. It is about cultivating long-term habits that support your hormonal health, boost your testosterone levels naturally, and ensure that your body functions optimally as you age.

1. **Balanced and Nutritious Diet**: Your diet plays a fundamental role in maintaining healthy testosterone levels. Nutrient-dense foods that provide essential vitamins, minerals, and healthy fats help promote the production of testosterone. Here's how to tailor your diet for optimal hormone health:
   - **Healthy Fats**: Testosterone is a fat-soluble hormone, which means it needs healthy fats to thrive. Incorporate monounsaturated and polyunsaturated fats into your diet by consuming olive oil, avocados, nuts, seeds, and fatty fish like salmon and mackerel. These fats

have been shown to support the body's ability to produce testosterone.

- o **Protein for Muscle and Hormone Health**: Lean protein sources, such as chicken, turkey, eggs, and legumes, are crucial for testosterone production. Protein is also important for muscle growth and repair, which plays a role in maintaining healthy testosterone levels, particularly as you age.
- o **Zinc-Rich Foods**: Zinc is an essential mineral for testosterone production. Foods like oysters, beef, spinach, pumpkin seeds, and cashews are rich in zinc and can help ensure that your body has enough of this mineral to support optimal testosterone levels.
- o **Vitamin D**: Low levels of vitamin D have been linked to lower testosterone levels. Sunlight exposure is the best source of

vitamin D, but you can also find it in foods like fortified dairy products, egg yolks, and fatty fish.

- **Vegetables and Fibre**: Vegetables, especially cruciferous ones like broccoli, cauliflower, and Brussels sprouts, contain compounds that can support testosterone production and help regulate oestrogen levels. Fibre-rich foods like whole grains, beans, and legumes help balance hormones and regulate blood sugar, which indirectly supports testosterone levels.

2. **Exercise and Physical Activity**: Exercise is one of the most effective ways to maintain or increase testosterone levels. The right type of physical activity can stimulate the body's natural production of testosterone and help improve other health factors such as cardiovascular health, muscle mass, and body composition.

   - **Strength Training and Resistance Exercises**: Lifting weights or engaging in resistance training is particularly effective at increasing testosterone levels. This type of exercise stresses your muscles, signalling to your body that it needs to produce more testosterone to repair and grow muscle tissue. Aim for at least two to three strength training sessions per week, focusing on compound exercises like squats, deadlifts, and bench presses that work multiple muscle groups.

- **High-Intensity Interval Training (HIIT)**: HIIT workouts, which alternate between short bursts of intense activity and recovery periods, are also effective in boosting testosterone levels. HIIT has been shown to increase testosterone production and improve metabolic health, cardiovascular fitness, and fat loss.
- **Consistency Over Intensity**: While intense exercise can boost

testosterone, excessive amounts of high-intensity training without adequate rest can have the opposite effect and reduce testosterone levels. Striking the right balance between exercise and recovery is crucial for long-term hormonal health. Be sure to incorporate rest days and lower-intensity exercises like walking, swimming, or yoga into your routine.

3. **Quality Sleep**: Sleep is perhaps one of the most underestimated factors in testosterone health. Your body produces testosterone primarily during deep sleep, so poor or inadequate sleep can have a significant impact on testosterone levels.

   o **Aim for 7-9 Hours of Sleep**: Most adults need between seven and nine hours of sleep per night to support hormonal health. During deep sleep stages, the body produces the highest levels of testosterone, which is essential for maintaining physical

health, mental clarity, and
emotional well-being.

○ **Establish a Consistent Sleep Schedule**: Going to bed and waking up at the same time each day helps regulate your body's internal clock, improving the quality of your sleep. This consistency allows your body to enter deeper sleep cycles, which are critical for testosterone production.

○ **Improve Sleep Environment**: Your sleep environment plays a significant role in the quality of rest you get. Keep your bedroom cool, dark, and quiet to promote uninterrupted sleep. Minimise exposure to blue light from screens (phones, computers, TVs) at least one hour before bedtime, as it can interfere with the production of melatonin, a hormone that helps regulate sleep.

4. **Stress Management**: Chronic stress is one of the biggest culprits in disrupting hormonal balance, and high stress levels are often associated with lower testosterone. When you experience stress, your body releases cortisol, a hormone that can suppress testosterone production. Learning to manage stress effectively is crucial for maintaining healthy testosterone levels.

   - **Mindfulness and Meditation**: Practising mindfulness, meditation, or deep-breathing exercises can help reduce cortisol levels and create a sense of calm, which allows your body to restore its hormonal balance. Aim for at least 10-15 minutes of relaxation techniques each day.

   - **Physical Activity for Stress Relief**: In addition to boosting testosterone, regular physical activity helps reduce stress and lower cortisol. Even a short walk or stretching session can work wonders for your mental state and hormonal health.

- ○ **Social Connections**: Engaging in positive social interactions and nurturing relationships with family and friends can help mitigate stress. Having a strong support network is vital for emotional well-being and balancing stress hormones.

5. **Avoiding Toxins and Hormone Disruptors**: Certain chemicals in our environment, such as endocrine-disrupting chemicals (EDCs), can interfere with hormone production and disrupt testosterone levels. These toxins can be found in plastics, pesticides, and personal care products.

   - ○ **Minimise Exposure to Plastic**: Bisphenol A (BPA), found in many plastics, is known to interfere with hormone levels and can negatively impact testosterone. To reduce exposure, use glass, stainless steel, or BPA-free plastic products for food and drink storage.

- ○ **Check Personal Care Products**: Many personal care products, such as shampoos, lotions, and deodorants, contain chemicals that can disrupt hormone balance. Choose natural or organic alternatives that are free from parabens, phthalates, and other harmful ingredients.

6. **Moderating Alcohol Consumption**: While a glass of wine or an occasional beer might not have a major effect on testosterone, excessive alcohol consumption can have a negative impact on hormone levels. Heavy drinking raises oestrogen levels, reduces testosterone production, and can impair the body's ability to metabolise fat.

   - ○ **Limit Alcohol Intake**: Moderating your alcohol consumption and avoiding binge drinking is essential for testosterone health. Stick to moderate drinking guidelines, such as one drink per day for women and two drinks per day for men.

7. **Maintaining Healthy Body Composition**: Testosterone production is closely tied to body fat percentage. Excess body fat, particularly abdominal fat, can lead to higher levels of oestrogen, which can suppress testosterone production. Maintaining a healthy body composition through proper diet and exercise can support your hormone levels.

   o **Focus on Fat Loss and Muscle Gain**: Incorporate both resistance training and cardio into your fitness routine to help reduce excess body fat and increase lean muscle mass. This combination supports healthy testosterone production and improves overall metabolic health.

Building Long-Term Habits for Hormonal Health

To achieve lasting testosterone health, it's important to commit to long-term changes that support hormonal balance. This requires consistency, patience, and the willingness to adapt to a healthier lifestyle. Here are some tips for building habits that support testosterone production:

- **Start Small and Build Gradually**: Trying to overhaul your entire lifestyle overnight can be overwhelming. Instead, focus on small, manageable changes that you can sustain over time. Gradually increase your physical activity, improve your diet, and implement stress-reducing techniques one step at a time.
- **Track Your Progress**: Keep a journal of your lifestyle changes and monitor your progress over time. Tracking things like sleep quality, exercise routines, and mood can help you identify patterns and make adjustments as needed.
- **Stay Accountable**: Find a workout buddy, join a fitness group, or share your goals

with a trusted friend or family member. Having someone to hold you accountable can keep you motivated and committed to your testosterone-boosting lifestyle.

Putting it All Together: A Sustainable Plan

A sustainable plan for maintaining testosterone health is about balance. It's not just about one aspect of your lifestyle but a comprehensive approach that includes proper nutrition, regular exercise, quality sleep, stress management, and healthy habits. By taking small steps and making gradual adjustments, you can build lasting habits that promote hormonal health and improve your overall well-being.

A testosterone-friendly lifestyle doesn't need to be extreme. It's about consistency and commitment to small, meaningful changes that support your body's natural ability to produce testosterone. In doing so, you will not only optimise your hormone levels but also improve your energy, mood, mental clarity, and physical

health—giving you a sense of vitality and
well-being for the long term.

Frequently Asked Questions About Testosterone

Testosterone, often called the "male hormone," is essential for a variety of bodily functions in both men and women. However, despite its crucial role in health, there are many myths and misconceptions surrounding it. As awareness of testosterone's importance grows, so does the number of questions people have about this vital hormone. In this section, we'll address some of the most common concerns and misconceptions about testosterone, including frequently asked questions regarding testosterone replacement therapy (TRT), supplements, diet, and more.

Common Concerns and Misconceptions

1. **"Testosterone is only important for men."**
   - **Answer**: While testosterone is commonly associated with male health, it is equally important for women. Both men and women have testosterone in their bodies, but in different amounts. In women, testosterone is produced in the ovaries and adrenal glands and is crucial for maintaining libido, bone density, muscle mass, mood regulation, and overall well-being. Low testosterone in women can lead to a variety of issues, including fatigue, mood swings, and reduced sexual desire.
2. **"Testosterone makes you aggressive."**
   - **Answer**: This is a common stereotype, but the truth is more nuanced. While testosterone can influence mood and behaviour,

there is no direct link between the hormone and increased aggression in the majority of people. Testosterone does play a role in assertiveness and competitiveness, but these traits do not automatically translate to violence or aggression. It's essential to note that aggression is influenced by a variety of factors, including environment, mental health, and upbringing, not just hormones.

3. **"Testosterone replacement therapy (TRT) is only for elderly men."**
   - **Answer**: While testosterone levels naturally decline with age, low testosterone can affect men of any age, not just older adults. Conditions like hypogonadism, where the body produces insufficient testosterone, can occur in younger men as well. TRT can be beneficial for those with clinically low testosterone levels, regardless

of age, but it should only be considered after thorough testing and a discussion with a healthcare provider. It's important to remember that TRT should be personalised and monitored regularly.

4. **"Testosterone causes hair loss."**
   - **Answer**: Testosterone itself does not directly cause hair loss, but an increase in the hormone can trigger hair loss in people genetically predisposed to male or female pattern baldness. This condition is related to dihydrotestosterone (DHT), a byproduct of testosterone. If you're concerned about hair loss while undergoing TRT or increasing your testosterone levels, it's important to consult with a doctor to discuss potential side effects and treatment options.

5. **"Taking testosterone is unsafe and has serious side effects."**

- o **Answer**: Like any medical treatment, testosterone therapy can have side effects. However, when used correctly under the supervision of a healthcare professional, testosterone replacement therapy (TRT) is generally safe. Potential side effects include fluid retention, acne, sleep apnea, and an increase in red blood cell count. Long-term or unsupervised use, especially in excess, can cause complications, but with proper monitoring and dose adjustments, these risks can be minimised.

6. **"Testosterone is only about muscle building."**
   - o **Answer**: While testosterone does play a key role in muscle mass and strength, its effects are far-reaching. It also impacts bone density, mood regulation, cognitive function, libido, and overall energy levels. Testosterone is essential for the

health of the heart, liver, and other vital organs. Its influence extends beyond just physical appearance, affecting both mental and physical health.

Answering Popular Questions on TRT, Supplements, and Diet

1. **"When should I consider getting tested for low testosterone?"**
   - **Answer**: If you're experiencing symptoms like fatigue, low libido, difficulty concentrating, mood swings, or unexplained weight gain, it might be time to check your testosterone levels. However, testing is often most beneficial when symptoms are persistent and interfere with daily life. Testosterone levels fluctuate throughout the day, so testing is usually done in the morning when

testosterone levels are highest. Consult a healthcare provider to determine if testing is appropriate for you.

2. **"What are the different types of testosterone replacement therapy (TRT)?"**
   - **Answer**: There are several forms of testosterone replacement therapy available, each with its own pros and cons. These include:
   - **Injections**: Testosterone injections are one of the most common methods. They are typically administered every 1-2 weeks by a healthcare professional or self-administered at home. The benefit of injections is their effectiveness, but some men experience mood fluctuations as testosterone levels rise and fall between doses.
   - **Patches**: Testosterone patches are worn on the skin and provide a

steady release of testosterone over time. They are easy to use but can cause skin irritation in some individuals.

- o **Gels and Creams**: Testosterone gels and creams are applied to the skin daily. They are a convenient option but may cause skin irritation or transfer to others if not applied correctly.

- o **Pellets**: Testosterone pellets are inserted under the skin by a healthcare provider and release testosterone gradually over the course of 3-6 months. While they are convenient and provide steady hormone levels, they require a minor surgical procedure for insertion.

3. **"Are testosterone-boosting supplements effective?"**

- o **Answer**: Testosterone-boosting supplements are widely marketed, but their effectiveness varies. Many supplements contain ingredients such as fenugreek, D-aspartic acid, zinc, and vitamin D, which may support healthy testosterone levels. However, the scientific evidence supporting the effectiveness of these supplements is often limited. In some cases, they can have a mild effect on testosterone levels in individuals who are deficient in certain nutrients, but they are unlikely to dramatically increase testosterone in healthy individuals. Always consult with a healthcare provider before starting any supplement regimen.

4. **"Can diet help increase testosterone levels?"**
   - **Answer**: Yes, diet plays a significant role in maintaining optimal testosterone levels. A balanced diet that includes healthy fats, protein, and essential vitamins and minerals can support

testosterone production. For example, foods rich in zinc (such as oysters, beef, and pumpkin seeds), vitamin D (from fatty fish, egg yolks, and sunlight), and healthy fats (like olive oil, avocados, and nuts) can help maintain healthy testosterone levels. Limiting processed foods, sugar, and excessive alcohol consumption is also important to support hormonal health.

5. **"How long does it take to see results from TRT?"**
   - **Answer**: The time it takes to see results from testosterone replacement therapy can vary. Some individuals may begin to notice improvements in energy, mood, and libido within the first few weeks. However, it can take several months for full benefits, particularly in terms of muscle mass and bone density. Regular follow-up visits

with a healthcare provider are essential to monitor progress, adjust doses, and address any side effects.

6. **"Are there natural ways to boost testosterone levels without TRT?"**
   - **Answer**: Yes, there are several natural ways to support and boost testosterone levels. These include:
   - **Exercise**: Regular physical activity, particularly strength training and high-intensity interval training (HIIT), can stimulate testosterone production.
   - **Healthy Diet**: Eating a balanced diet rich in nutrients such as zinc, vitamin D, healthy fats, and protein can help maintain testosterone levels.
   - **Sleep**: Getting 7-9 hours of quality sleep per night is crucial for hormone production, including testosterone.
   - **Stress Management**: Chronic stress leads to high cortisol levels,

which can suppress testosterone. Practising relaxation techniques such as meditation, yoga, or deep breathing can help lower stress and support testosterone health.

- o **Weight Management**: Maintaining a healthy weight is important for balancing testosterone levels, as excess body fat can lead to lower testosterone production.

7. **"What happens if I don't treat low testosterone?"**

- o **Answer**: Untreated low testosterone can lead to a variety of health issues, including decreased libido, fatigue, mood swings, depression, and cognitive decline. Over time, low testosterone can also lead to a loss of muscle mass, increased body fat, and bone thinning, increasing the risk of osteoporosis and fractures. Additionally, low testosterone levels have been associated with an increased risk of cardiovascular diseases. Treating low testosterone can help alleviate these symptoms and improve overall quality of life.

8. **"Can TRT be stopped after starting it?"**

   o **Answer**: Testosterone replacement therapy is a long-term treatment that is usually continued indefinitely. If therapy is stopped, testosterone levels will likely drop back to their previous low levels. However, if TRT has been effective, your body may produce some testosterone naturally again. In some cases, doctors may try to reduce the dosage or switch to different treatments. Always consult with your doctor before stopping any form of TRT to understand the potential effects and determine the best course of action.

9 798345 955277